Assessment and appraisal of doctors in training

Principles and practice

Edited by

George Cowan FRCP

Medical Director, Joint Committee on Higher Medical Training,
Royal College of Physicians
Formerly Dean, Postgraduate Medicine, North Thames Deanery

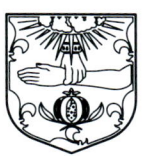

Royal College of Physicians

Royal College of Physicians of London
11 St Andrew's Place, London NW1 4LE

Registered Charity No 210508

ISBN 1 86016 132 4

Typeset by Dan-Set Graphics, Telford, Shropshire
Printed by Sarum ColourView Group, Salisbury, Wiltshire

Foreword

All doctors in training after full registration are now required to be *assessed* regularly against criteria devised by their respective specialties and based on the qualities of a doctor as set out by the General Medical Council in *Good Medical Practice*.[1] This assessment is usually conducted by a consultant who is in overall charge of the training of the junior doctor – with external input when necessary. However, fair and open judgements cannot be made without the support of a framework of *appraisal* of doctors in training by their trainers. Both trainees and trainers require to be educated in the correct methods of conducting these processes.

The Royal College of Physicians has recently published a new generic curriculum for senior house officers in medical specialties and an appraisal record to support it.[2] The curricula for higher specialist training in all medical specialties are also being rewritten within a framework designed to enhance the rigour of the assessment of specialist registrars. It is therefore timely that this book should appear to support these initiatives. It gives insight and guidance into the processes of assessment and appraisal and provides a valuable resource both for consultants in all specialties involved in the training of junior doctors, and for specialist registrars who are preparing for their consultant responsibilities.

May 2001

KGMM Alberti
President
Royal College of Physicians

1. General Medical Council. *Good Medical Practice*. London: GMC, 1998.
2. Royal College of Physicians. *Core Curriculum for SHOs* (3rd edn) and *Personal Training and Appraisal Record for SHOs*. London: RCP (in press).

About the authors

George Cowan

Formerly Dean of Postgraduate Medicine for North Thames Deanery, with special responsibility for medical and psychiatric specialties and for appraisal and assessment across North Thames. He is a physician with a special interest in gastroenterology and tropical medicine, and is now Medical Director of the Joint Committee on Higher Medical Training at the Royal College of Physicians.

Maurice Greenberg

Consultant Psychiatrist at University College London Hospitals NHS Trust and Head of Student Counselling Service at University College, London.

Peter Mills

Consultant Cardiologist at the London Chest Hospital, Chair of the Specialty Training Committee for Cardiology in North Thames East, and Vice-Chair of the STC in General Internal Medicine in North Thames.

Elisabeth Paice

Dean Director of Postgraduate Medical and Dental Education for North Thames since 1995, and for London since April 2001. Previously Consultant Rheumatologist at Whittington Hospital, where she was also Clinical Tutor (1990–1993). Co-opted member of the Council of the National Association of Clinical Tutors (since 1993). Represents COPMeD on the BMA Education Board. She has published on the educational problems of the senior house officer grade, charters and logbooks for pre-registration house officers, disillusioned doctors, the impact of Calman and other educational topics.

Edward Rosen

Appointed Education Adviser for North Thames West in 1993, with responsibility for training senior registrars and consultants in assessment, appraisal and annual review skills. In 1995 appointed Education Adviser for North Thames with responsibility for delivering appraisal training across the region. Has held positions in higher education at Oxford, Portsmouth and New

cont.

York, where he contributed to curriculum planning and innovation. He was appointed a member of the NHS/CCSC Working Group on Appraisal, and of the British Association of Appraisal Managers.

Isobel Williams

Consultant Physician in Respiratory and General Medicine at St Albans and Hemel Hempstead NHS Trust, and Chair of the Specialty Training Committee in General Internal Medicine in North Thames.

Contents

Glossary

BMA	British Medical Association
CCST	Certificate of Completion of Specialist Training
CMO	Chief Medical Officer
COPMeD	Council of Postgraduate Medical Deans
GIM	General internal medicine
GPT	General professional training
JCHMT	Joint Committee on Higher Medical Training
MRCP	Member of the Royal College of Physicians
NTN	National training number
PRHO	Pre-registration house officer
PYA	Penultimate year assessment
RITA	Record of in training assessment
SAC	Specialist Advisory Committee
SHO	Senior house officer
SpR	Specialist registrar
STA	Specialist Training Authority
STC	Specialty Training Committee

1 Appraisal and assessment: definitions

George Cowan

Medical Director, JCHMT, Royal College of Physicians

> Happiness at work depends on *being fit for it* [assessment], *not having too much of it* [the New Deal], *a sense of success in it* [appraisal]
>
> John Ruskin, 1851

> *Life is short and the art long*
>
> Hippocrates

A central element of the Calman reforms in the training of hospital doctors in 1993 was the introduction of the regular *assessment* of progress, within structured training programmes of defined length and content, for the specialist registrar (SpR) grade. At the same time, it was recognised that good educational progress towards successful episodes of assessment, introduced to protect the public against badly trained specialist doctors, must be facilitated by regular confidential meetings of the trainer and trainee to provide feedback and to agree new training goals. This process is now called *educational appraisal*. The terminology has since become (or has remained) confused, and it is essential that certain working terms be universally agreed.

Educational appraisal

To carry out educational appraisal, the trainee and trainer should meet privately and confidentially on a regular basis to provide opportunities for:

▶ reflective self-appraisal by the trainee;
▶ constructive feedback from the trainer, both positive and negative;
▶ mutual agreement of the next set of training goals and objectives, and their context;
▶ the production of a written summary of the plan which has been mutually agreed (which of itself need not be confidential); and

▶ arrangement to meet again to review progress made and set new goals.

These structured private meetings complement – but do not replace – traditional episodes of informal or immediate on-the-job feedback during ward rounds, outpatient clinics, operating and endoscopy lists.

Perhaps unfortunately in a semantic sense, educational appraisal can also be called *formative assessment*, and is so called in the monitoring of training of general practitioners. It is essentially a developmental tool, employing regular feedback from the trainer, but also involves certain set testing methods (eg review of videotaped consultations with patients).

Summative assessment

The process of *summative assessment* involves regular episodes of formally reviewing doctors' performance in training against minimum standards of progress defined for each specialty by the Specialist Training Authority and the Royal Medical Colleges. This is a regulatory judgemental process, which depends on the production of auditable written evidence of performance drawn from a range of sources:

▶ reports from trainers of the attainment of the necessary knowledge and practical skills;
▶ assessment by the trainers and other health professionals of the behaviour of the trainee in personal attributes such as good communication, professional integrity and commitment;
▶ written or computer-based examinations or tests;
▶ simulated practical skills tests;
▶ observation against structured criteria of professional activity (eg record-keeping, ward rounds, outpatient clinics, surgical operations, endoscopy, etc); and
▶ personal development plan records and learning portfolios which also contain evidence of activity in research, audit, formal teaching and learning, and personal reflection.

> **Educational appraisal** of doctors in training should *not* therefore be regarded as:
>
> ► summative assessment
> ► regulatory
> ► punitive
> ► a form of counselling (for which a different setting, context and counsellor may be desirable)
> ► a job interview
> ► affecting pay and promotion.

Evidence of the positive effects of good educational appraisal on the perception by doctors of the value of their training posts is provided in Chapter 4.

Performance appraisal

Performance appraisal (or performance review) is a tool of management and not primarily an educational process, although it should contain elements of personal development planning. Performance against personal and organisational objectives is reviewed in a confidential interview, and new goals are set for both contexts. This process is widely used in industry and government. If properly conducted, it should usually be a positive experience for the subject, although it may be constructed so as to have an effect on promotion and job progress.

Performance appraisal is *not* applied to doctors in training, but is – or will be – the basis of the 'appraisal' of *consultants* in hospital practice and their *personal development* plans.

Record of in training assessment

The process by which a panel of consultants (*not* including the trainer) from the same specialty as the trainee SpR review the *evidence* of progress against the standards set by all Royal Colleges is known as the record of in training assessment (RITA). It is not in itself an assessment, but leads to a decision as to whether or not the trainee may progress to the next stage of training, and with what additional training goals. It could be argued that this process should be called a *review* of in training assessment. A similar regular process for the review of the progress of senior house officers is being developed.

Summary

The two processes of *educational appraisal* and *summative assessment* of doctors in training are thus separate but interdependent (Fig 1 and Table 1). A fair assessment of the trainee cannot be made by a trainer who has not regularly, honestly and openly apprised that trainee of all the positive and negative aspects of his/her performance and progress. The appraiser and the chief assessor are most often, but not necessarily, the same consultant, a consultant who will know most about the trainee professionally and as a person. The required detached judgement of progress should be made annually by the RITA panel, which provides the trainee, the postgraduate dean and the Royal College concerned with a final decision. Both processes should provide mechanisms to remedy any deficiencies which may be agreed in appraisal or defined by assessment. The summative assessment system must be open to formal appeal.

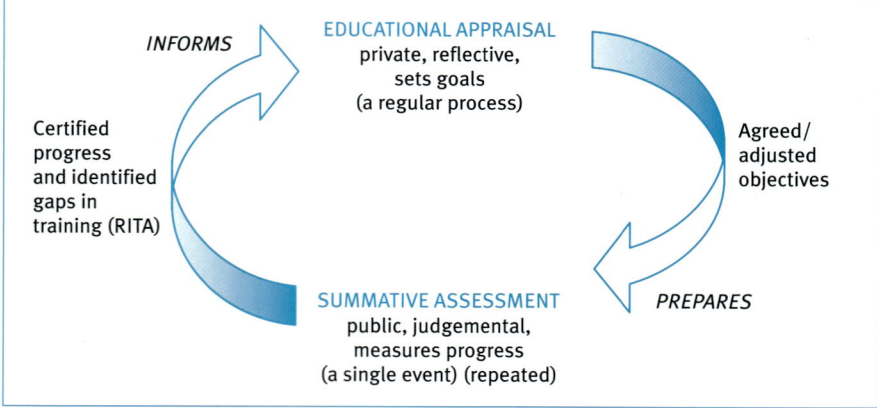

Fig 1. *The interdependence of educational appraisal and summative assessment* (RITA = record of in training assessment).

Table 1 Appraisal, assessment and review: summary of definitions

Educational appraisal	Summative assessment	Record of in training assessment
Regular (*at the start, in the middle and at the end of a training post*)	Annual (*usually*)	Annual
Developmental	Judgemental	Regulatory
Local	Local	Regional or supra-regional
Confidential discussion	Open documents & records	Review of trainer's reports & training records
Agrees new objectives, results in personal development plan	Compiles training records against national standards (*may include examinations*)	Decides normal progress or remediation based on written evidence
Performed by educational supervisor	Performed by educational supervisor, unit training director or training programme director	Performed by deanery panel*

* The deanery panel comprises the chair of the specialty training committee, two or three consultants in the specialty (not including own appraiser or assessor), and may include an external reviewer (eg from specialist advisory committee).

2 Principles of good practice in appraisal

Edward Rosen

Education Adviser, Department of Postgraduate Medical Education (North Thames), University of London

In the recently published report, *Supporting doctors, protecting patients,*[1] appraisal is defined as:

> A positive process to give someone feedback on their performance, to chart their continuing progress and to identify development needs. It is a forward looking process essential for the development and educational planning needs of an individual.

This definition of appraisal is one which is widely accepted amongst professionals engaged in developing appraisal systems in different organisational contexts. Appraisal is generally accepted as providing opportunities for individuals to reflect critically on their performance in the workplace and to identify their personal development needs.

An indicator of high quality in appraisal is that it is a skilled conversation between a trained appraiser and an appraisee (trainee doctor). In many professional contexts appraisal provides an opportunity for an individual to align his/her personal and professional learning objectives with the broader objectives and needs of the organisation in which he/she is employed.

Principles of good practice in appraisal

A good place to start discussing appraisal is to focus on the principles underpinning good practice in appraisal. Many of these principles first emerged in the business sector, and have been adapted and refined in other professional sectors (eg teaching, law and nursing). The following principles are presented as a contribution to the discussion about an appropriate appraisal system for the medical profession as it contributes to the modernising agenda in the new NHS.

The ten principles

1 Appraisal systems take *time to be successfully implemented* within an organisation. Appraisal systems cannot be introduced without successfully engaging all those directly involved in implementing the system. All appraisal systems that have been introduced as a top-down initiative have tended either to collapse within three to five years or have evolved into a formalistic bureaucratic ritual of ticking boxes – and have therefore become meaningless as human developmental activity.

2 *Appraisal is not assessment.* The process of appraisal should be clearly understood and recognised as separate from the assessment of competence and/or progress in training:

   ▶ *Appraisal* should be understood as a professional activity which seeks to support the individual appraisee's development over a period of time.
   ▶ *Assessment* seeks to make professional judgements on the level of competence of the individual against recognised public standards, referred to in Royal College curricula.

3 Appraisal should be *integrated into the professional relationship between the appraiser and appraisee.* An appraiser should be someone who has a supervisory or monitoring role in relation to the appraisee. Consultants with direct responsibilities for supervision and monitoring should be considered as potential appraisers.

4 All individuals concerned with managing the appraisal process must be trained to do so competently. Good quality appraisal systems are those in which there has been initial *training and development of appraisers and appraisees.* Appraisal systems that have ignored this principle have usually degenerated into unproductive meetings of little benefit to either the appraisees or the organisations in which they are employed. It is worth emphasising that even committed, enthusiastic appraisers will periodically need opportunities for further training in order to gain new insights in their roles as appraisers. An appraisal system that offers continuing opportunities for reflective practice for appraisers is better able to contribute to change management.

5 A high performance appraisal system is one in which *appraisers are encouraged to reflect on their skills and competencies* in their roles as appraisers as part of their own professional development. Good appraisal systems enable appraisees to reflect on their performance in

the workplace and provide opportunities for them to engage in a process of self-appraisal, which is one element of professional self-regulation in action.

Trainees who take part in training workshops should be taught how to take responsibility for managing their self-appraisal. This is not a difficult skill to learn. *Self-appraisal* as a principle should therefore contribute to ways in which 'individuals take responsibility for the quality of their own practice'.[2]

6   *Documentation* should be as simple as possible. Appraisal should not be primarily a paper-led exercise or lead to production of endless paper (see principle 9). It is primarily an educational activity informed by appropriate and relevant documentary evidence which could include:

▶ a self-appraisal form prepared by the trainee;
▶ an agenda for the appraisal meeting written by the appraiser; and
▶ any other relevant written documentation previously agreed by both appraisee and appraiser.

7   It is an essential principle that the appraisal discussion is *confidential.* Appraisal meetings are private conversations between two individuals which should be held on the basis of honesty, mutual trust and respect. Anything spoken about during the appraisal meeting should not be discussed with any other person without the trainee's explicit permission. Appraisal conversations should be structured and provide formal opportunities for appraisees to review their personal and developmental needs in an atmosphere of support and encouragement. These meetings should be non-threatening and as friendly and relaxed as possible. They should take place as often as required to enable the appraiser to give constructive feedback to the appraisee. During a one-year rotation it is suggested that there should be a minimum of three meetings over the year.

8   Appraisal meetings that might be interrupted by bleeps, incoming telephone calls and other distractions are likely to fail. *Time should be set aside* to ensure that the meeting is uninterrupted. It should be timed to enable a thorough review of all the items identified on the trainee's self-appraisal form, and planned with adequate time set aside for the discussion to take place in an atmosphere which is unhurried and unpressured.

We have found that good appraisal discussion usually takes 30–60 minutes. This seems to be the norm in most appraisal systems. When the appraiser and appraisee are experienced in the process of constructive dialogue it is likely that the discussion will achieve all its objectives in a reasonable amount of time. Less experienced colleagues may take longer to master the process. The level of experience of both parties engaged in appraisal should be taken into consideration when planning the first appraisal meeting.

9   The meeting should result in an *agreed written document*. This is likely to be a personal development plan. The CMO has recently written that:

> Personal development plans will form part of the appraisal cycle and will help direct an individual's continuing personal development.[3]

The outcome from an appraisal meeting should be a personal development plan which is signed by the two parties as representing a consensus on the development needs the trainee has identified. It is also evidence that an appraisal meeting has taken place.

The PDP should not contain more than four or five objectives to be achieved by the appraisee during a rotation. The plan could become an important document in the individual's professional portfolio or progress file, as evidence of progress and achievement in the training programme.

10   Finally, the *trainee assumes ownership* of the process and takes responsibility for maintaining records of appraisal meetings. As the trainee moves from one post to another, the documentary evidence from appraisal should be available for initial appraisal meetings with new trainers.

References

1 Department of Health. *Supporting doctors, protecting patients: a consultation paper on preventing, recognising and dealing with poor performance of doctors in the NHS in England.* London: DoH, 1999.

2 *Ibid*: page 55, 5.1.

3 *Ibid*: page 60, 5.17.

3 Educational appraisal: process and practice

Maurice Greenberg

Consultant Psychiatrist, University College London Hospitals NHS Trust

A wise man learns from history, a foolish man learns from experience.

Chinese Proverb

The appraisal of a junior doctor in training differs from that of a consultant in a number of ways. Perhaps the most emotive is that a trainee will always be appraised by a senior colleague. It is essential that someone with greater experience, who is in a position to support their professional development carefully, assumes this responsibility. In order to ensure that appraisal works as effectively as possible, it must be clearly demarcated from issues of general management. Trainees are only too well aware that they depend upon personal support for their progress. For appraisal to be useful, the trainee needs to believe that it is undertaken in their interests; it is therefore essential that they develop trust in their appraiser.

Although the focus of this book is on trainees, it might be nice to think that the general principles outlined below would apply just as well to consultant appraisal. However, in this situation the establishment of trust is possibly even more complicated, since suspicion about their relationship with whoever appraises them may be inevitable. The process of appraisal has been borrowed from the world of business, where hierarchies in management are much more clearly defined than in medicine, although they apply more closely to a training model. One way to help overcome this difficulty would be to offer consultants a choice over who appraises them.

Junior doctors have to absorb an enormous number of facts during their training, acquire considerable clinical skills, and learn how to apply these thoughtfully in their work as independent professionals – all complicated and time-consuming tasks. Given the considerable amount of knowledge they have to acquire, there is a danger that they will simply learn to regurgitate facts without enquiring into their usefulness. I firmly believe that the capacity to reflect and think should be encouraged and developed in doctors. This is more likely to occur if they learn to ask thoughtful questions about themselves, their practice and their environment. If appraisal is approached from this perspective, a form of curiosity which encourages doctors to question themselves as much as others can be nurtured.

The definition of appraisal that I follow, 'a review of progress against agreed objectives', seems fairly uncontentious and straightforward, but in order to establish a framework for appraisal it is essential to understand the context within which it takes place.

Context of appraisal

Three considerations shape what takes place during an appraisal:

1 Who is doing the appraisal?
2 At what stage of training is the person who is being appraised?
3 What is the trainee's job description?

Who is doing the appraisal?

The context of appraisal is determined first by the professional relationship between the person undertaking the appraisal and the recipient. This is important because what happens will depend upon whether the senior person involved is, for example, the trainee's consultant, their specialty tutor or a postgraduate dean. In practice, their consultant is much more likely to be interested in detailed 'hands-on' issues, such as specific clinical skills, whereas their specialty tutor is more likely to take a broader view of the trainee's overall training needs.

At what stage of training is the person who is being appraised?

An appraisal will differ depending on whether it is for someone embarking upon a first post-registration job or for an almost fully trained individual who anticipates becoming a consultant in the near future. In the first case, the appraiser will need to be much more active in setting out the framework and planning what takes place, and should expect to have some objectives to offer the trainee. On the other hand, I would expect a more experienced specialist registrar to be much clearer about what needs to be focused on, and would be rather disappointed if they did not come up with any ideas of their own. Part of the educational process ought to include the trainee assuming increasing responsibility for shaping his or her own appraisal.

What is the trainee's job description?

The realistic opportunities for training that will be available should be clearly specified in the job description, and will be influenced by whether the post is independent or part of a rotational scheme. In the former case, it is more likely that training will be specifically determined by the particular post, and that appraisal will focus on the individual's progress within it. In the latter situation, a broader view of development and training is likely to emerge during appraisal, and will probably be undertaken by someone for whom the trainee is not working. The details of the job description will also determine what can be achieved by, for example, clarifying the time constraints and the specific opportunities on offer.

Planning appraisals

All the above implies that a considerable amount of planning needs to take place before an appraisal meeting. I think it is unrealistic to ignore the appraiser's contributions at the meeting, even though they may say little. It is therefore essential that appraisers recognise their responsibilities and skills in this situation.

The following five aspects need to be considered when planning appraisals:

1 Frequency
2 Setting
3 Content
4 Style
5 Records.

Frequency

One simple rule about how often an appraisal should take place is that there must be at least three meetings:

▶ *The first meeting*: agreed objectives should be set out, how they will be evaluated, and what help will be needed to meet them;
▶ *At least one interim meeting* to allow progress to be monitored in order to see whether the objectives were realistic and the support offered sufficient;
▶ *The final meeting*: a review of overall progress.

The actual number of meetings will depend on how long the individual is in a particular post or on a particular rotation. If the appointment is for six months, three meetings will probably be sufficient; if longer, then about three meetings a year may be needed.

When this appraisal system was set up for the first time in our trust, some of us forgot the interim meeting, and discovered that the objectives were being set at the beginning and the review was taking place at the end of the trainee's placement. If things were going well, there were no problems, but if progress was unsatisfactory nothing much could be done when it was only pointed out at the final meeting. If an appraisal takes place too frequently it loses its impact. However, it is helpful to maintain informal contact from time to time to find out how the trainee is progressing.

Setting

The meeting needs to take place in a comfortable setting at a time set in advance. Depending upon the context, I think at least one hour will be needed to do justice to the discussion, although views may vary about this (eg see Chapter 2). It is helpful to introduce the framework and some ideas before the meeting, either with a brief discussion, or a note, or both, spelling out the general aims and inviting the trainee to think about it for him- or herself.

It is essential that there are no interruptions during the meeting and that there is a total focus on the appraisal. Junior doctors are bound to be anxious about sitting down with a consultant or a tutor. Talking about problems over working hours, or even potential disciplinary matters such as time-keeping, will be distracting and unsettling. The sort of mistake it is only too easy to make is to suggest to your junior doctor, whom you were intending to appraise later in the week, that you might as well do it now because you both have a spare half hour.

Content

Although the aim is to encourage a junior doctor to produce his or her own agenda, it is essential that the appraiser has a view about what topics should be raised. The worst scenario is not finding anything to talk about, and either having an uncomfortable silence or ending the interview early.

One advantage of thinking about it beforehand is that it allows consultants to clarify what they would like a trainee to learn from working with them, which is easier in some specialties than in others. Someone who has applied to a specific rotation or for a particular post ought to have some idea of what they want to achieve from it. However, the agenda is potentially unlimited, and could include anything from a desire to acquire a particular clinical skill to learning how to work with difficult colleagues. In the introductory briefing, it can be helpful to outline some of the topics that the junior doctor could talk about. The skill of appraisal is to help the trainee recognise, or discover for themselves, what they would like to achieve and what help will be required. When this has been clarified, the consultant will be in a position to offer appropriate support. It is essential, however, to have realistic aims. For example, there is no point in promising a trainee the opportunity to attend a particular course when their timetable will not allow this.

It is necessary to remember that appraisal cannot be undertaken in ignorance of the trainee's general progress. For example, the trainee may have a particular problem with time keeping. If they fail to address this, the consultant must do so.

Finally, do not overdo it; there should not be an enormous number of objectives – in my view, three are sufficient. Individuals are much more likely to succeed if their aims are realistic; it is a fact that if people show progress in one area, and appreciate it themselves, there is an associated halo effect.

Style

It is impossible to legislate for style. I recognise that not everyone can be like me – it may even be possible that not many would want to be! It is therefore essential for trainers to accept their own style and to work within it. However, being positive always helps. A senior colleague at UCL described to me how, during his gap year, he taught science in the sixth form at his school. He was given one of the weaker classes to teach, and decided that he would compliment them for anything they achieved. They produced the best results of the year. I believe this story, but know how difficult it can be to put things positively. One of the reasons we find it difficult to say things in a positive fashion is because it takes longer. It is easier and quicker to say, 'That was a mistake, don't do it again', than to say, 'I can see why you did this. However, if you tried it this way it might have been much more effective'. This requires practice, but making the effort does pay off; it enables people to listen, and to learn, much more effectively.

Records

When the objectives have been agreed, it is useful to write them down and confirm them with the trainee. It can be helpful to send the trainee a note confirming the details, partly because it is easy to forget verbal arrangements and partly because it provides some record of their (and your) consistency and development. Many training schemes now use log books and, provided it is kept simple, an appraisal can be incorporated into these (see Chapter 4).

Support

It is essential to have some training in appraisal. If this can be provided collectively for a group of colleagues who work together, it helps them develop a shared view about what they are trying to achieve and how they want it to be undertaken. It also allows them to come up with general principles and to offer ongoing support to each other – this is necessary because appraisal is both time-consuming and challenging.

Conclusion

Thinking about these general points can help facilitate the appraisal process, but it must be remembered that it will not resolve every problem that arises, nor compensate for a poor training programme, nor sort out the difficulties created by poor trainees. It can, however, help clarify what underpins these situations. Faults in a particular placement should become apparent, and can then be addressed. Similarly, weaknesses in an individual trainee should be revealed, which might be due either to inappropriate career choice or to personality characteristics. The former can be helped through career counselling, but the solutions to many of these situations lie elsewhere and cannot be achieved through appraisal alone.

4 Appraisal as part of the training experience: perceptions of trainees

Elisabeth Paice

Dean Director, Postgraduate Medical and Dental Education for London

Feedback is an essential element in learning. Without this, it is difficult for learners to know when they are getting things right or wrong. In medicine, the tradition has been for the consultant supervisor to give trainees immediate feedback when things went wrong, but to take what they did right for granted. Silence was expected to be taken as approval, or at least as absence of disapproval. This approach fell into disrepute in the early 1990s as organisations outside medicine recognised the importance of feedback and introduced regular performance appraisal against agreed performance objectives. In education, the concept of appraisal was also gaining momentum, and the University of London made it a compulsory feature of all its posts in 1993. Various reports from those involved in postgraduate medical education also recognised the importance of appraisal in training, and recommended educational objective-setting at the start of each post with regular feedback on progress toward those objectives during the course of the placement. Regular one-to-one confidential discussions between trainee and consultant supervisor were recommended by postgraduate deans and Royal Colleges alike. It seemed likely that these appraisal sessions would improve the quality of the training experience, thus improving job satisfaction and perhaps even reducing stress.

This chapter considers evidence accumulated within the North Thames Region that the essential elements of appraisal – that is, educational objective-setting and subsequent discussion of progress with a supervising consultant – improve the experience for doctors in training.

The pre-registration house officer log book

In 1989, the postgraduate dean for South-East Thames suggested introducing a log book for pre-registration house officers (PRHOs). It would, he hoped, 'by developing feedback and evaluation, create a spirit of "glasnost" between juniors and seniors'. He recommended that the log book should:

▶ clarify the educational aims of the PRHO year;
▶ provide a check-list for both seniors and juniors;
▶ record career counselling; and
▶ provide a tool for monitoring and assessing achievements.

He also recommended that the trainee should have the opportunity to record his or her opinion of the post, the trainer and the training, to be shared with the clinical tutor and the educational supervisor.

This stimulated the first concerted effort to introduce appraisal for doctors in training in North Thames. The first version of the log book was produced in 1991. It contained check-lists for:

▶ self-assessment of practical procedures performed;
▶ emergencies experienced; and
▶ educational topics covered.

It also contained advice for the consultant about how to set objectives at the beginning of the post and offer structured feedback at intervals thereafter.

An evaluation exercise in 1994 showed that house officers who discussed the log book with their consultant were significantly more satisfied with their induction, consultant supervision, formal and informal education, and feedback than others, and more likely to recommend their post. As one house surgeon said:

> I was a bit disappointed with my job. I didn't think I had done enough – procedures and all that. Then my consultant went through the list of things in the log book with me, and I realised how much I had learned. It was quite surprising. I felt a lot better about the job.

The survey suggested that time spent by consultants in planned, well-structured discussions with their house officers about their problems and their performance was an important factor in enhancing the educational value of the PRHO year. The log book appeared to be a useful tool for adding structure and focus to such discussions.

Appraisal and senior house officers

When the postgraduate deans tried to implement appraisal for senior house officers (SHOs), there was scepticism among consultant trainers about its value. Many consultants found it embarrassing or artificial to sit face-to-face with a trainee and talk about their performance, nor were they keen to have their own performance as trainers discussed. Some consultants considered such discussions unnecessary, since day-to-day interchange made it clear what they thought of the trainee's performance – they let the trainees know quickly enough if they were not satisfied.

A survey by the postgraduate deans of SHOs in all specialties in North Thames in 1992-93 revealed that only 35% had sat down with their consultant to talk about their progress, even after three months or more in post. Those who had done so were significantly more likely to give a good rating to their consultant supervision and to recommend their post than those who had not. This evidence, fed back to the consultants, did much to change attitudes. A similar survey of SHOs in the same hospitals two years later demonstrated that 48% in post for over three months had had a useful discussion about their progress with their consultant.

Appraisal training

Starting in 1993, the postgraduate deans began to organise appraisal training sessions for consultants, usually taking the form of one- or two-day interactive workshops, with role play and videos. Some specialties, notably paediatrics, took a particular interest in developing documentation to provide trainees and trainers with a framework to support the educational dialogue. In addition, the Royal Colleges, universities, the National Association of Clinical Tutors and other bodies began to offer courses. When the Calman reforms of specialist training were introduced in 1995, educational objective-setting and regular feedback on progress were to be required features of every specialist registrar (SpR) post. This further stimulated interest in appraisal training, and by 1998 it was estimated that approximately a third of consultant supervisors in the region had received training in appraisal.

The North Thames trainee surveys

A great deal was learnt about appraisal and its impact on the educational experience of trainees from two major questionnaire surveys carried out during and after the implementation of the Calman reforms (1996–97 and 1998–99, respectively). These covered all grades, all specialties and all training hospitals and community trusts, and together yielded 6,358 responses (response rate 74%).

The questions explored satisfaction with the educational quality of the current post and included two questions relevant to appraisal:

1 Did you discuss your educational objectives with your consultant at the beginning of this post?
2 Have you sat down with your consultant to discuss your progress in this post?

The phrase 'sat down with' was used to exclude the sort of brief, unplanned and opportunistic discussions that might take place walking down the corridor or in theatre. We avoided the term 'appraisal' as it was not universally understood by trainees. We offered a *yes/no* response to each of these questions, but in the case of the consultant discussion of progress question this was modified to:

▶ Yes, and it was useful.
▶ Yes, but it was not useful.
▶ No, but it was not necessary.
▶ No, but it will happen.
▶ No, but I would have liked to.

Most of the other questions required the trainee to indicate their satisfaction with various elements of their training using a five-point scale (1 = very poor; 5 = excellent).

Educational objective-setting

In the first survey (1996–97), 50% of trainees reported having discussed their educational objectives at the start of their current post. By the second survey (1998–99), the figure had risen to 62%. The more senior the trainee, the more likely this discussion was to have taken place. Objective-setting was most likely to have occurred in the psychiatric specialties and was least likely in the surgical specialties, with the medical specialties in between. In all grades and specialties, and in both surveys, educational objective-setting was associated with significantly higher ratings for most aspects of training, especially:

▶ induction;
▶ consultant supervision; and
▶ satisfaction with the job as a whole.

Discussion of progress with consultant

The design of the study was such that, at the time of each survey, a proportion of trainees would have started their posts too recently to have discussed progress with their consultant. However, we would expect these trainees at least to know such a discussion was planned. In the first survey, 37% of trainees reported having had a useful discussion with their consultant about their progress, while another 20% knew that such a discussion was planned. Two years later, 42% had had a useful discussion, and 27% knew a discussion was planned (Fig 1).

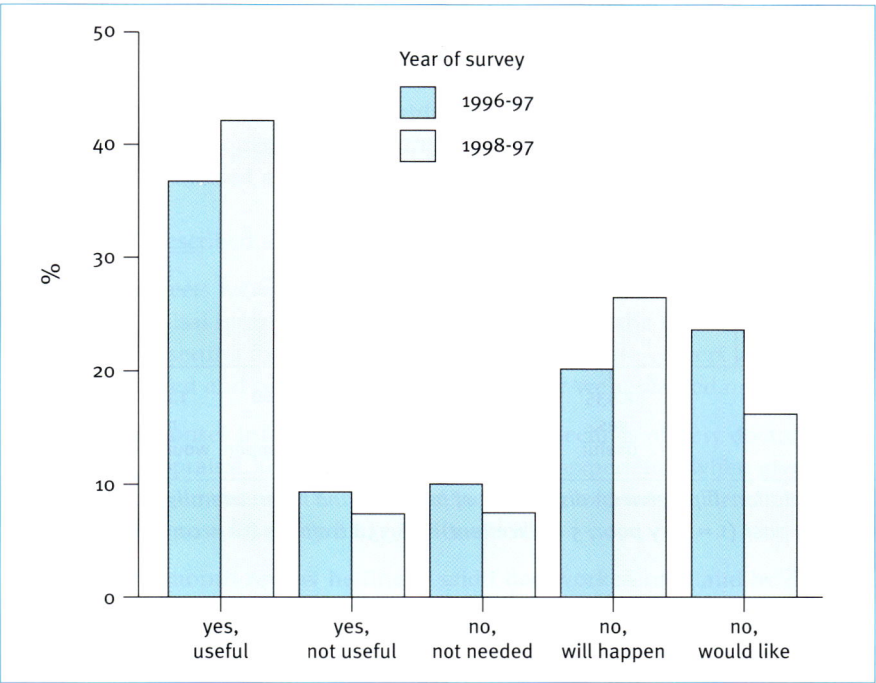

Fig 1. *Responses to the question 'Have you sat down with your consultant to discuss your progress in this post?'* (Surveys of trainees 1996–97 and 1998–99).

Although many consultants had dismissed as unnecessary the idea of formally sitting down to offer feedback, only 10% of trainees in the first survey and 7% in the second chose the response 'No, but it was not necessary'. Differences between the specialties were most marked at SpR level, where the proportion of trainees reporting having had useful feedback ranged from 63% in accident and emergency medicine to 27% in anaesthetics. Medical specialties were again in the middle of the range at 45%. Those who had discussed their educational objectives with their consultant at the beginning of the post were nearly three times as likely to report useful feedback. There was a strong correlation between having had useful feedback and high ratings for induction, hands-on experience gained in the post, and consultant supervision. The relationship between the responses to this question and overall satisfaction with the post is illustrated in Fig 2.

medicine do you get told when you do well, but only when you do wrong! Felt – ecstatic!'

Conclusion

Evidence provided by trainees indicates that appraisal improves the training experience. Time spent by a consultant in offering a structured, positive educational dialogue is highly prized and motivating for the trainee, whereas ill-prepared, poorly timed and negative feedback can have devastating consequences. Appraisal is a skill that needs to be learnt and regularly practised if its potential benefits are to be realised.

References

1 King RC. A log book for pre-registration house officers. *Br J Hosp Med* 1989;**41**:111.
2 McManus IC. From selection to qualification: how and why medical students change. In: Allen I, Brown P, Hughes P (eds). *Choosing tomorrow's doctors*. London: Policy Studies Institute, 1997.
3 Paice E, West G, Cooper R, Orton V, Scotland A. Senior house officer training: is it getting better? *Br Med J* 1997;**314**:719–20.
4 Paice E. Why do young doctors leave the profession? *J R Soc Med* 1997;**90**:41–2.
5 Paice E, Moss F, West G, Grant J. Association of use of a log book and experience as a pre-registration house officer: interview survey. *Br Med J* 1997;**314**:213–5.
6 Paice E. Is the New Deal compatible with good training? A survey of senior house officers. *Hosp Med* 1998;**59**:72–3.
7 Paice E, Aitken M, Cowan G, Heard S. Trainee satisfaction before and after the Calman reforms of specialist training: questionnaire survey. *Br Med J* 2000;**320**:832–6.

5 Principles of assessment of doctors in training

George Cowan

Medical Director, JCHMT, Royal College of Physicians

> *Assessment is an essential element of all structured training programmes*
>
> Calman Report, 1993[1]

The regular assessment of the progress of specialist doctors undergoing structured training is one of the central requirements of the Calman reforms in medical training. General practitioners in training had for some years previously been subject to a single summative assessment episode to certify their fitness to practice as a principal. Specialist registrars (SpRs) in programmes of up to six years of training were judged to require an annual summative assessment which would determine their fitness to proceed in training or identify additional educational needs.

Regular assessment of all junior training grades is not yet fully established. Systems to assess pre-registration house officers in the two, three or four posts held in the year before full registration are now being put in place. Some specialties have yet to impose formal assessment systems on senior house officers (SHOs) – the exceptions are anaesthesia, obstetrics and gynaecology, and surgery. Steps are now being taken to make this applicable in all specialties, and for a review process to be developed similar to the record of in training assessment (RITA). Generic documentation for RITA for SHOs is being developed.

Summative assessment

Purposes

The summative assessment of SpRs has three objectives:

1 The protection of patients and the public from badly trained doctors.
2 The documentation of the professional development of trainees.
3 The justification of the expenditure of public money on the training of doctors.

Characteristics

Summative assessment should have the following characteristics:

1 It is formal, judgemental, open, honest and documented, with the full knowledge of the trainee as to methods and criteria.
2 It regularly (usually annually) measures progress against external standards laid down by the Royal Colleges in curricula and sets of competencies under the supervision of the Specialist Training Authority, the body which advises the General Medical Council on the admission of specialist doctors to the specialist register.
3 It provides written evidence, which can be substantiated or challenged, of appropriate progress in knowledge, skills, professional behaviour, and attitudes of the trainee.
4 It should be reliable, valid in content, acceptable to assessors and trainees, predictive in value, non-discriminatory in respect of gender, race, origin, etc, and cost-effective.
5 It is compiled by the sharing of judgements by consultant trainers and non-medical colleagues (a process known as triangulation).
6 It should have positive effects on the educational progress of trainees, and thus be acceptable to them.

Methods

The available methods used in summative assessment, which are best used by combining different methods in parallel, include:

1 Trainers' reports on professional knowledge, preferably referenced to written curricula and criteria.
2 Directly observed performance review, for example, case notes, ward rounds, outpatient clinics, surgical and other practical skills, with the possible addition of videotaped patient interviews.
3 Written judgements of behavioural characteristics, for example good communication with patients and colleagues, integrity, commitment, leadership of teams, good appreciation of the objectives of the NHS and the trust, preferably incorporating views from other consultants, senior nursing staff, managers, etc.
4 Criterion-referenced reproducible examinations and tests, for example multiple choice questions, observed structured clinical examinations, modified essay questions, viva.
5 Documented evidence of other educational endeavour in cumulative personal development plans or learning portfolios, for example audit, research, publications, presentations, learning courses, teaching and reflection.

Problems with summative assessment in practice

In practice, there are a number of problems with summative assessment:

1 Lack of training of assessors by their Royal College or postgraduate dean.
2 Lack of clear criteria, competencies, documentation and standardised assessment methods, which are the responsibility of the Royal Colleges.
3 Lack of data on educational and clinical outcomes, and hence of evaluation of the process.
4 Lack of case law regarding defensibility, fairness and non-discrimination.
5 Concerns over indemnity for assessors. This is covered largely by Health Service Circular 1999/015, which provides that doctors acting in this respect for the postgraduate deans will be indemnified by the Department of Health, provided that they follow deanery procedures and do not break the law with regard to unlawful discrimination.
6 Confusion of the process with appraisal by trainers, trainees and other bodies, both in terms of terminology and training.
7 Issues about the transfer of information, in that:
   ► the trainee must be told in writing what information is being transmitted to a new trainer or trust;
   ► the information must be factual;
   ► patient safety must be paramount;
   ► educational needs need to be addressed educationally, and not in a disciplinary fashion and, conversely;
   ► disciplinary problems and health issues should be addressed appropriately.

Prevention of problems in assessment

Many problems in the training of doctors and the assessment of their progress can be avoided by the following procedures:

1 The training of assessors and their commitment with that of their trainees to the process.
2 High quality personalised induction, both written and verbal, on matters such as protocols, rotas, timetables and training opportunities.
3 An early objective-setting meeting with the educational supervisor (otherwise called the first appraisal meeting), resulting in an agreed plan for training enshrined within a personal development plan.
4 Ongoing regular educational appraisal of good quality and value.

5 Consultant supervision leading to graduated responsibility based on observation of competence, judgement and behaviour.

6 The consultant supervisor acting as a good role model.

7 Clinical practice within the team or unit or hospital based on evidence-based medicine and general integrity.

8 Regular summative assessment based on good appraisal and good evidence.

Record of in training assessment

A record of the annual review, and therefore of the SpR's progress through his or her training programme, is provided by RITA. It is normally completed annually by members of the specialty training committees under the aegis of the postgraduate dean. In some specialties, at different points in the training, this review panel is attended by an external reviewer from the Specialist Advisory Committee.

RITA is not in itself a means of assessment. The function of the RITA review is to determine whether the trainee may pass on to the next stage of training (or has completed it) or requires additional remedial training, which is specified and made known to the trainee, and to the next training consultant and NHS trust. It is a process which must be open to review and appeal, but should also be capable of determining that a trainee is so deficient that removal from the training programme should be recommended and can be defended. It is important to note that it is not normally materially influenced by personal factors which may have delayed training (eg illness) which need to be dealt with on their own merits. It can be argued that RITA should be retitled a *review* of in training assessment, the assessment having been carried out by the trainee's own trainer or training programme director. It is therefore important that the assessor in that context should not be a member of the RITA panel so that the panel can be as objective as possible.

Practice currently varies between specialties and between deaneries in respect of the personal involvement of the SpRs under review. In small specialties and small deaneries the trainee will almost invariably be present every time his or her progress is reviewed. However, this becomes a very large logistic exercise in big specialties and deaneries, and some specialties have made the case that, at least in some years of training, the documentary evidence provided of satisfactory progress will be regarded as acceptable. In these circumstances, the SpRs should be given the option to attend in person if they wish. Otherwise, the RITA panel will make a judgement 'on paper' if no difficulties are perceived in the trainee's progress. Where problems are anticipated from the written reports, it is not uncommon for additional members of the panel to be added, even sometimes including postgraduate deans themselves (postgraduate deans should not normally attend RITA panels but keep themselves in reserve for appeal hearings).

Problems with the record of in training assessment

Problems are reported with the conduct of the RITA process both by trainees and by the panels themselves:

1 Sometimes there is a lack of notice to the panel or the trainee, or both, and a lack of administrative support.

2 In some cases there is clearly confusion of the process with:
   ▶ assessment itself (of the trainee, the post or the trainer);
   ▶ negotiation of, or selection for, the next post;
   ▶ career advice;
   ▶ counselling;
   ▶ a job interview; or
   ▶ an appeal court.

3 The presence of the doctor's own trainer is likely to lead to a lack of objectivity and openness in the process but, conversely, an opaque, dishonest or bland trainer's report creates difficulties in itself.

4 Trainees may allege that any problems perceived by the trainer have not been fed back to them in appraisal meetings, or the trainee may challenge the quality or quantity of the training itself.

5 Some trainees complain of a punitive atmosphere or an impression that the process is a *viva* examination and not a review of their assessment.

6 Documentation provided by the Royal Colleges may vary in quality, the trainer may not have filled in the documents properly, or the trainee may not have taken appropriate responsibility in seeing that this happens.

7 Where untoward clinical incidents or unprofessional behaviour are described in assessment reports there is often lack of written evidence of such episodes. This evidence is essential if appeals are to occur.

8 Recipients of form E in the RITA process which delays their Certificate of Completion of Specialist Training date may subsequently claim prejudice and disadvantage in their new training placement. This will be in a new environment, and they feel distrusted, under the spotlight and not provided with sufficient clinical responsibility. Form E

placements also raise the issues of resources in that it is often necessary for the postgraduate dean to place them in a supernumerary placement, with extra time and responsibility for their trainer and the possibility of additional risk to patients. These issues require to be carefully negotiated with the new trainer and trust.

Reference

1 Department of Health. *Hospital doctors: training for the future.* (The Calman Report). London: DoH, 1993.

6 Record of in training assessment: review in practice in the medical specialties

Peter Mills

Consultant Cardiologist, London Chest Hospital

Isobel Williams

Consultant Physician, Respiratory and General Medicine, St Albans and Hemel Hempstead NHS Trust

In medical subspecialties, the general internal medicine (GIM) component of training and the subspecialty itself need to be assessed. These two components are generally best assessed by different members of the Record of In Training Assessment (RITA) panel.

Trainees commonly need to be reminded of the need to describe their GIM training experiences. This is best achieved by 'open' questions such as 'tell us about a patient/or audit subject outside your specialty from which you gained useful lessons'. The subspecialty assessment will in the first instance be based on the report from the local educational adviser. Discussion of training objectives should be structured around the Joint Committee on Higher Medical Training (JCHMT) curriculum booklet. Educational supervisors and members of RITA panels must be familiar with the contents of the subspecialty and the GIM curricula.

The paperwork

The RITA process serves to keep the trainee, the deanery and the Royal College in touch with progress through the training programme. The paperwork involved in this process has the prime objective of documenting the progress (or lack of progress) through an appropriate programme. The training record is the possession of the trainee until a certificate of completion of specialist training (CCST) has been awarded, when it will be available to the Specialist Advisory Committee (SAC) and may be audited by the Specialist Training Authority (STA).

As trainees become accustomed to the concept of a training record, their ability to keep this up-to-date and completed improves. Most trainees who entered the specialist registrar (SpR) grade after 'transition' on 1st January 1997 have adapted well to the process which, currently, may be regarded as being *in lieu* of an exit examination. Nevertheless, the individual character of the trainee is invariably reflected in the degree of completeness and tidiness of their record, and their ability to present the record as an aid rather than a hindrance to critical evaluation.

The RITA panel needs to have an accurate and current knowledge of both the SAC's curriculum requirements and the achievements thus far of the trainee. Constructive shaping of the future training programme for the individual will minimise the chance of irredeemable problems being encountered when the external SAC representative attends the penultimate year assessment (PYA) meeting:

- *RITA Form A* ensures that the deanery has access to current demographic information, address, telephone and e-mail of the trainee.
- *RITA Form C* ensures that the year under assessment has been completed to the satisfaction of the RITA panel.
- *RITA Form D* or *Form E* indicates specific (D) or general (E) dissatisfaction with the trainee's progress. Before issuing these verdicts, the panel will wish to liaise with the deanery and the training directors about the consequences of this action.

Structure of the assessment

A minimum of three assessors is required. The time required varies with the quality of the trainee; 15–30 minutes (average 20 minutes) is usually appropriate. We have found it helpful if one member of the committee summarises the panel's recommendations for the following year.

Entry to the training programme

The entry criteria will now usually have been addressed by the SpR appointment committee. These include:

1 At least two years in the senior house officer (SHO) grade, with 18 months dealing with emergency admissions (which may be in subspecialties) and six months unselected general medical takes.
2 Experience in 'registrar' posts prior to MRCP cannot be recognised as training contributing to CCST.
3 Experience in senior SHO posts after MRCP cannot be recognised as training contributing to CCST.
4 General professional training outside the UK can be recognised only by prior agreement with the JCHMT office.

Higher medical training

In the medical subspecialties, GIM is usually included in dual accreditation. Single specialty training lasts four years, GIM three years, and a dual accreditation training programme a total of five years. In cardiology, the training time is six years.

The GIM component of dual accreditation currently occurs in the early and later years of training (normally the first year and the last two years), but changes to deliver most, if not all, GIM training prior to subspecialty training are being considered.

Time spent in research can count towards one of the training years in the subspecialty, but not in general medicine. However, for trainees who already hold a national training number (NTN), one clinic monthly and one on-call per month (for one year) can be aggregated to a total of two months training. Thus, over a period of three years, a trainee could accumulate a total of six months GIM. This is the maximum accreditable time permitted through this mechanism.

The training record (the 'grey book')

Many trainees experience difficulties in coming to terms with the training record. Section 7 of the training record is designed to document specific activities throughout the length of higher medical training, and the annual RITA meetings provide the ideal time to review these issues:

1 Attendance at locally organised teaching sessions, as well as national and international meetings, should be documented. The RITA panel can discuss with the trainee whether or not sufficient formal education is occurring.
2 Research presentations and publications should be documented. This part of section 7 should be read in conjunction with the research supervisor's reports in section 8.
3 The trainee should document teaching commitments in section 7.
4 Advance life support course certificate should be filed in section 7.

The process

1 Appraisal at the beginning, middle and end of each training post by the educational supervisor.
2 Local assessment, which may be carried out by the educational supervisor or unit training director and filed as the educational supervisor's report in section 8 of the training record.

Local

Educational supervisor

The supervisor should be a consultant whose name appears on the Specialist Register.

The supervisor should be appointed by the deanery specialty training committee.

Every trainee should have a named supervisor(s) in each rotation post of a training programme. The trainee should be notified in writing of the name(s) of this person or persons.

Where the supervisor is absent for one reason or another for a period in excess of four weeks, another educational supervisor should be appointed with the approval of the responsible individual at deanery level.

Supervisors may delegate certain training modules to non-consultant career grade doctors in appropriate circumstances, but they retain overall training responsibility.

Although trainees can, and do, gain valuable experience when working in conjunction with other junior staff, the overall responsibility for training remains with the supervisor.

There are situations where non-medically qualified persons may act as educational supervisors for part of the training on the authority, and with the approval, of the programme director or equivalent person. This would tend to occur in specialties such as psychiatry, pathology and nuclear medicine, but may be used in other specialties.

Supervisors should liaise with others in the supervision chain where difficulties are experienced in the trainee achieving their educational objectives.

Supervision

The educational supervisor should ensure that the trainee receives adequate and appropriate clinical and managerial supervision during his or her training. Such supervision may be provided by the educational supervisor but may alternatively be provided by other appropriately qualified practitioners.

The level of such supervision required at the time will necessarily depend on the competence and experience of the trainee.

The closeness of clinical supervision should be at one of four levels:

1 direct (eg in the consulting room or at the operating table with the trainee);
2 nearby (eg in the theatre suite or outpatients department);
3 in the hospital and available; or
4 outside the hospital and available.

No trainee should be required to assume responsibility for, or perform, unsupervised clinical, operative or other techniques for which they have insufficient experience and expertise. Trainees should perform tasks without direct supervision only where both they and the supervisor are satisfied regarding their competence to do so. Both trainees and supervisors should at all times be aware of their responsibilities for the safety of patients in their care.

The educational supervisor should be in regular contact with the trainee. At the early stages of training this should be for at least one session per week, though in the later stages less frequent contact would be appropriate.

The educational supervisor should ensure the delivery of a particular component(s) of training as detailed in the curriculum.

There should be continuing appraisal, with trainee involvement and feedback.

The supervisor should be aware of the mental and physical well-being of the trainee and take action where appropriate.

The supervisor should ensure that the trainee receives appropriate career and other guidance.

The supervisor should facilitate and encourage attendance at educational programmes.

The supervisor should check that any problems in respect of communication or medical ethics are overcome.

The supervisor should check that the trainee's clinical, technical, administrative and organisational skills are developing as appropriate.

The supervisor should help with both professional and personal development and ensure that the trainee is not overburdened by clinical commitments, on the one hand, or underexposed, on the other.

If the performance is not reaching the required standard, the matter should be discussed with the trainee and remedial measures put in place as soon as possible.

Regional/deanery supervision

Postgraduate deans are responsible for the management and delivery of all medical postgraduate training carried out in the NHS and grant 'dean's staffing approval' to placements; this approval confirms that a training placement is of an acceptable standard, that trainees are supervised and that they assume clinical responsibilities compatible with their progress in training.

There are deaneries in all parts of the UK. A named person at deanery level should have responsibility for the supervision of training, and each trainee should be informed in writing of the name of this person. It is important that such a person should have been appointed or approved by the postgraduate dean in consultation with all the interested parties (eg local consultant body, specialist advisory committee and/or College higher training committee).

National

Specialist advisory committee

The specialist advisory committee (SAC) has the overall responsibility of supervising accredited posts and programmes, and trainees in a given specialty.

Joint higher training committees

These bodies, when present, have the overall responsibility of supervising the work of related SACs.

Colleges and faculties

These have overall responsibility for supervising the working of the higher training committees and SACs, if applicable.

Statutory body

The STA is the UK's statutory competent authority responsible for supervising all medical training at senior house officer (SHO) and specialist registrar (SpR) level intended to lead to the award of a CCST.

Higher specialist training structure

Table A.1 shows the direct line of responsibility from the trainee (SpR) to the STA. It does not list all those with an involvement in specialist training nor does it reflect training at SHO level.

Table A.1 Direct line of responsibility from the trainee to the Specialist Training Authority

Line structure	Others
Trainee (Specialist Registrar)	
Educational supervisor	
	College tutors
Programme director	
Specialty training committee	Regional specialty training adviser
SAC or JCHT (where applicable)	Postgraduate dean
College/faculty	
STA	